Start Sleeping With Your Wife Again

A Practical Sex Life Guide For Men in Sexless Relationships

Adam Lewis

Introduction

Remember when you couldn't keep your hands off each other? Those early days when a quick drive for takeout felt like foreplay, and eye contact across a crowded bar made your blood pumping? The sexual tension was so thick you could cut it with a knife—pure electricity.

But then, what happened? Life had other plans than supporting your sex life.

Suddenly, you're juggling:
- A mortgage that demands attention
- A career that takes more than it gives
- Family expectations from all directions
- Changes in your body and energy levels
- Stress that seems never to clock out
- A bedroom that's become more a sleep sanctuary than a love nest

Maybe you're wondering where things shifted. When did your sex life become an occasional thought? When did it all start feeling like a distant memory?

This book isn't about blame or shame. Your situation? It's more common than you think. Relationships evolve, and sometimes sex takes a backseat. It doesn't mean you've failed, and it doesn't mean you can't reignite that flame.

It isn't about quick fixes. It's about understanding what's happening and taking meaningful steps to rebuild your sex life. I'm here to give you honest, practical strategies that work in the real world.

Throughout the following chapters, we'll cover everything you need to start having sex with your wife/girlfriend again. I will show you what turns a woman on, how to bring back that spark, become a legendary lover, and much more.

My goal with this book is to make sex a regular thing in your relationship again, even if you haven't had sex in years, the kids are always in the way, or something else is blocking you and your lady from getting wild in the sack. I hope I'm able to deliver that to you.

Ready to stop thinking about how good things used to be and prepared to start making it even better?

Chapter 1: The Raw Truth About Dead Bedrooms

I overheard something in a Manhattan bar last month that stopped me mid-drink.

This guy at the end of the bar – in an expensive suit, probably in his early forties, beaming that Wall Street energy – was getting honest with the bartender after his fourth whiskey.

"Six hundred and forty-three days," he said, fidgeting with his wedding ring. "That's how f*cking long it's been since my wife has touched me. I mean really touched me. Like, 'I need you inside me right now' touching."

He laughed, but the kind of laugh that makes you question if a person is okay. "Want to hear the truly pathetic part? I got it logged on my phone. The exact date. What kind of man keeps track of how long his wife hasn't wanted him?"

I looked around that bar. Friday night in Midtown: packed with suits loosening their ties, most of them probably thinking they're different. I wondered how many of those guys went home to women who'd rather watch "Love is Blind" than sleep with them. How many lay in bed next to their wives, both pretending to be absorbed in their phones, trying to remember what good sex felt like?

The real gut punch? This wasn't some basement-dwelling troll. A tailor-made suit that likely costs more than most people's rent, fresh cut, and a Rolex on the wrist. Some partner downtown. At least, he was on paper, crushing life. In his bedroom? Crickets.

Maybe you're not at six hundred days, but you know something is wrong. Want to know the truth about why sex life dies?

Here's the thing most relationship "experts" won't tell you: sexual attraction isn't about physical appearance or bedroom technique. Sure, letting yourself go doesn't help, but the real killer of attraction runs deeper than your beer gut or receding hairline. It's about the slow, almost invisible transformation from the confident, ambitious man she couldn't keep her hands off to the comfortable, predictable guy who's become more of a roommate than a lover.

The good news? You can turn this ship around. Bad news? It's going to take more work than buying flowers.

First up is communication. Most guys would prefer a root canal than have an honest discussion about why their woman isn't attracted to them anymore. They dance around the issue, try to guess what's wrong, or worse, act like everything is okay while silently resenting their partner. Don't do that.

You need to have that uncomfortable conversation. And by uncomfortable, I mean it needs to be raw and real. No holding back, no sugar-coating, no defensiveness. Ask her straight out: "When did things change between us? What turned you on about me in the beginning? What's missing now?" Then comes the hard part: listening.

When women talk about losing attraction, a couple of patterns emerge.

One of the biggest killers? Emotional distance. Women get turned on by feeling connected. That doesn't mean you must become a sensitive poet who cries at sunset. It means being present and engaged in your relationship. Remember when you first started dating? You actually listened to her stories, asked questions, and shared your thoughts and dreams. Now, are you half-listening, thumbs scrolling down your phone, grunting occasionally just to fake it like you are listening? If so, stop doing that.

This quickly leads to the comfort trap.

Getting comfortable in a relationship isn't a bad thing per se, but there's this thin line between comfortable and complacent. Too many guys cross that line without even knowing it. You stop making an effort in your appearance, your conversation becomes limited to household logistics and complaints about work, and your idea of excitement is ordering from a different takeout place.

Meanwhile, you're wondering why she's no longer ripping your clothes off.

Next up is neediness, the attraction kryptonite.

Are you constantly needing validation, asking if she still finds you attractive, or getting hurt when she's not in the mood? Women are attracted to men with their own stuff going on;

they bring value to them instead of just taking it. I'm not saying you should be rude, but you do need to have a life apart from your relationship. So, hobbies, goals, and friendships.

Now, for the physical part.

Yes, it does matter. I'm not saying you must have washboard abs or look like a male model. But you do need to have self-respect for your body and health.

If you carry around an extra thirty pounds, are always tired, and get exhausted walking up a flight of stairs, you are impacting more than just your looks. It affects energy, confidence, and hormones.

Low testosterone is the silent killer of relationships, turning men into moody, passive shadows of their former selves. Get your testosterone levels checked. Start moving heavy weights. Fix your diet. Sleep enough. These aren't just health tips but the bare minimum you should be doing.

Your mental game is just as important as the physical.

Intelligence and competence are powerful attractors. When was the last time you learned something new? Do you intellectually challenge yourself or have a serious conversation about something?

Women are turned on by men who can stimulate them intellectually. Men with passionate interests and informed opinions. Read books. Develop skills in things that interest you. Be someone worth having a conversation with.

Another essential quality is leadership.

When I say leadership, I don't mean being bossy, dictatorial, or using force. I mean taking the lead, having a vision for your life, and being proactive in your relationship. Stop waiting for her to call all the shots. Stop asking permission to do what you want with your life. Opportunities for excitement and adventure start flowing when you create them. Women find men hot who can lead without being jerks about it.

You also don't need to be rich but financially smart.

How you handle money reflects your ability to plan, take responsibility, and create security. If you're always broke, making impulsive purchases, or avoiding financial obligations, that's a huge turn-off. Create a budget. Set financial goals. Show you can think beyond immediate gratification.

The power of genuine appreciation can't be overstated.

When was the last time you actually noticed something specific about your partner and let her know about it? Something more than the generic "you look nice" but rather an actual observation of something she does well or something unique about her?

Most guys stop paying attention once they've "got the girl." They take their partner for granted, assuming she knows she's appreciated—a big mistake. The key here isn't empty flattery. Women can smell that a mile away. It's about genuine, specific appreciation expressed regularly.

Now, about the bedroom itself.

If your sex life has died, that's on you as much as it is on her. Too many guys approach sex like it's a transaction X, Y, and Z, expecting result A. Natural attraction doesn't work like that. You build up a vibe of excitement, tension, and trust. That means learning to read her body language, being patient, building anticipation, and, above all, making her feel safe to express her desires.

Remember, attraction is not about looks, money, or status. It's all about energy, presence, and authentic masculine power. It's about being the kind of man who knows his worth, lives purposefully, and brings real value to his woman. The sort of man unafraid to see hard realities and do the work necessary for positive change.

Stop making excuses. Stop waiting for things to get better magically.

Next, Let's look at what turns a woman on.

Chapter 2: What Really Turns a Woman On?

"Put your hand up if you're absolutely certain — and I mean bet-your-life certain — that your woman isn't faking it."

That's what I asked a room full of 200 men at a relationship seminar a few months ago. Know how many hands went up? Three. Most men shifted uncomfortably in their seats.

But it was the third guy that got my attention. Built like a linebacker, tattoos crawling up his neck, looking about as comfortable at a relationship seminar as a priest at a strip club. He wasn't laughing. Just sat there with his hand raised, dead serious.

After the talk, I pulled him aside. "What makes you so confident?" I asked.

His answer? "Because the first time she actually came with me, she started crying. Not fake tears – real, messy, mascara-running-down-her-face crying. Said she'd been faking it with every guy she'd ever been with for twenty years. Didn't even know what a real orgasm felt like until that night. Now? Now I couldn't get her to fake it if I tried."

Many couples live in a world of miscommunication and unfulfilled desires, where partners go through the motions while mentally drifting to their to-do lists or household tasks.

Let's have an honest conversation about pleasure and connection. Many partners aren't experiencing the fulfillment they desire, either because they're unsure about their needs or trying to protect their partner's feelings. If you're reading this, you might sense something's missing in your intimate life.

Perhaps the passion has faded, or your partner seems disconnected during intimate moments.

Here's the encouraging part.

Women are usually open about their needs and desires. They want genuine connection and pleasure. Let's look at what turns women on.

First, let's kill a common myth once and for all: guys are horndogs, and women need romance novels and scented candles. Male and female brains light up precisely the same when they see something hot. Women are just as sexual as men; they just express it differently.

The National Library of Medicine found both men and women hit their peak horniness at the same time watching porn-10 minutes flat. So, If there's a disconnect, it's usually about approach rather than capacity for pleasure.

Getting your lady turned on isn't a one-size-fits-all manual. Some women get turned on at the thought of danger, the threat of getting caught, perhaps playing strangers in a bar, or fooling around where you might get busted. The adrenaline makes everything more intense. It's the same chemicals flooding your system. The brain can't tell the distinction between the excitement of almost getting caught and the excitement of some good foreplay.

Others need to feel protected and safe, like they're in their private bubble where they can let go completely. They need to feel genuinely wanted. That means getting yourself together and handling her emotional needs before you even think about having sex with her.

Let's look at what works, starting with the foundation: genuine attention and active listening.

Real active listening means actually hearing what she's saying, not just head-nodding while you're thinking about something else. She needs to know you care about what's in her head. This is about creating the kind of bond that leads to intimacy. When she feels heard, she feels connected. And when she feels connected, she gets turned on. Next time she's talking with you, pay attention and listen.

Also, consider the impact of daily stress. Women's brains are like a computer with fifty tabs open. It's dishes, laundry, kids' schedules, and all the other life events that need doing. Do you want her thinking about being with you instead of the unwashed dishes? Then handle some of that stuff yourself. When your woman sees you taking initiative in managing life's demands, it creates space for her desire to grow.

Master the art of eye contact, not that creepy serial killer stare, but real, intimate eye-gazing. Two minutes, no talking. Feel awkward? Good. That's where the magic happens. This is some tantric sex-level stuff that works.

Low-hanging fruits: Try some real hugging with full-body contact. Massage her neck and hold her hand while walking, during dinner, or watching TV. Make it natural and frequent.

Want to really get her motor running? Get her adrenaline pumping. Excitement mimics arousal. Hit up some roller coasters, horror movies, or anything that gets the blood flowing. Science proves it. Couples who do crazy stuff together are more intimate because your brain associates that excitement with each other, creating a chemical cocktail that turns you both on. Also, the excitement of doing new stuff together creates shared experiences and inside jokes, and that spark in her eyes when she looks at you like she did on day one.

Here's another fun fact that will blow your mind. On average, women think about sex nineteen times per day. One out of three admitted to having kinky thoughts they wanted to try but feared being judged. So, create a space where she feels safe telling you her dirty thoughts. Maybe she wants to be tied up, maybe she wants to tie YOU up. You won't know unless you ask. Most guys are so focused on their fantasies they never even consider that their woman might have some wild ideas of her own.

What you can do tonight: grab a bottle of wine, sit down, and make your Yes/No/Maybe lists together. A study found that even long-term couples don't know what their partner hates in bed. Fix it. Write it all out: kinks, positions, fantasies, hard limits. Be honest about what gets you going and what doesn't. It's not just about knowing what new tricks you can try; it's also about avoiding those things that turn her off completely. Nothing kills the mood quite as much as crossing a boundary you didn't know existed.

As a fundamental truth, great sex has nothing to do with having a huge tool or memorizing the Kama Sutra. It has to do with creating the kind of relationship where she wants to rip your clothes off. It's about building tension, creating connection, and making her feel like the sexy goddess she is.

Chapter 3: How to Increase Her Low Sex Drive

Let me tell you about my boy Ron. I found him in the gym last week, staring in the mirror like it owed him money. His story hit close to home – it might hit close for many of you reading this.

It was another night when his wife, Kim, gave him a cold shoulder. Another night of him lying there with his dick in his hand while she's got her face buried in TikTok with her AirPods in, acting like he's not even there. Brutal.

Ron's 35, decent-looking dude, got his shit together, mostly. But this isn't how he thought married life would look like. Six years ago? These horny lovers were like teenagers who discovered their genitals for the first time. Couldn't leave them alone in a room without them trying to break some furniture. Kitchen counter? Done. Shower? Daily. He even told me about when they almost got caught banging in their garage during the neighbor's cookout.

Now? His bedroom's got all the sexual energy of a tax audit.

Sure, he's got a bit of a dad bod creeping in – who doesn't after years of marriage? But that's not the real issue. His girl Kim? She's getting railroaded by life. She got that fancy VP promotion eating her soul 60 hours a week.

Two kids with more activities than a cruise ship schedule. Her parents call with their geriatric emergencies every other day. The same chick who used to send him titty pics during board meetings now passes out before she can finish an episode of "Real Housewives" or whatever basic reality show she's watching.

Here's where it gets real. Last week, after another night of lying there like a monk, my boy finally cracked.

"Are we okay?" he asks, probably expecting the usual bull.

But Kim? She hits him real: "I miss us too." Then she dropped this bomb: "I just feel like I'm drowning most days. By bedtime, there's nothing left of me. Nothing. My sex drive is almost non-existent."

The same woman who used to blow him in the back row of movie theaters just because she was bored – now she's so drained she can't even find the energy to take care of herself.

And here's the thing that's messing with him – it's not even just about having sex anymore. He misses his partner in crime. Misses that crazy glint she'd get in her eye before doing something wild. Misses the woman who could make him hard and his heart full simultaneously.

I could see it in his eyes when he told me all this. My boy was done, hoping tomorrow would be different. He needed fundamental change.

That conversation was a wake-up call. Their problem wasn't lack of love – life was getting in the way. And maybe, just maybe, that meant there was hope. Because while you can't force desire, you can create the conditions where it naturally flourishes. This is how to do precisely that.

When your woman's sex drive vanishes, it feels like someone pulled the emergency brake on your relationship. Before you spiral into thoughts of her losing interest or eyeing other men, understand this - female desire is a complex beast, governed by a delicate dance of hormones, emotions, and physical factors. Even a rough day at the office can throw the whole system into chaos.

Think of her hormones like a finely tuned orchestra. When everything's in harmony, the music flows perfectly. But one wrong note - usually stress - and the whole symphony is ruined.

Estrogen leads the hormonal orchestra as the queen bee, working alongside testosterone (yes, women need it too), cortisol (the stress hormone), progesterone (keeping moods stable), and thyroid hormones (running the metabolic show.) When stress crashes the party, cortisol spikes and tells all these other hormones to take a hike.

Speaking of stress, it's time to wear your detective hat and figure out what's killing her vibe. It could be work drama, kids driving her nuts, money worries, family bullshit, or health issues. Your job isn't to fix everything but to be part of the solution. Take some weight off her shoulders. Handle more kid duty. Do the mental heavy lifting she's been carrying.

Create stress-free zones in your life together. Set up a weekly date night and stick to it. Make the bedroom a phone-free sanctuary. Ban work talk after dinner. Give her real alone time.

Now, about supplements. Some of this stuff actually works wonders. Maca root can kick the libido into gear naturally. Ashwagandha kills stress and supports testosterone. Vitamin D deficiency is a silent sex drive killer, and most women are running low. Magnesium helps with sleep and stress, while B-complex vitamins provide crucial energy and hormone support. But here's the catch: supplements are like putting premium gas in a car with engine problems. You've got to fix the underlying issues first.

Your diet choices can make or break your sex life. Load up on healthy fats like avocados, olive oil, and nuts. Get quality protein from wild-caught fish and grass-fed meat. Add complex carbs like sweet potatoes and quinoa, dark chocolate with at least 70% cocoa, and plenty of leafy greens for minerals and blood flow. Meanwhile, kick processed sugar, excess booze, too much caffeine, and shitty oils to the curb. These troublemakers wreck hormone balance, kill libido, spike anxiety, and cause inflammation.

Exercise matters too, but you've got to be smart about it. Start simple with daily thirty-minute walks together. Suggest yoga for better blood flow everywhere. Light strength training naturally boosts testosterone, and dance classes can help her feel sexy again. Don't push too hard - marathon training or daily HIIT workouts when she's already stressed might backfire spectacularly.

Your woman's biggest sex organ isn't between her legs - it's between her ears. Her brain needs as much attention as her body, maybe more.

Start with stress management. Practice deep breathing together, schedule regular massage sessions, and give her actual time to decompress. Not the kind where she's still thinking about a million things, but real, uninterrupted relaxation.

Body image plays a massive role, too. Your job isn't to fix her self-image - it's to make her feel desired and appreciated. Give specific compliments throughout the day. Touch her without expecting it to lead to sex. Create an environment where she feels safe and accepted, not just wanted for her body. Make her feel sexy as hell, but do it authentically.

When you make it to the bedroom, treat it like a five-star experience, not a fast-food quickie. Take your sweet time with foreplay. Learn to read her signals like a master detective. Don't rush straight to home base, pressure her, bring up past experiences, or sulk if she's not in the mood. That guaranteed to dry her up.

This isn't a quick-fix situation. You might see small changes in her stress levels in the first couple of weeks. Give it a month or two, and her hormone balance should improve. Real, significant changes in sex drive usually take three to six months. After six months of consistent effort, you'll establish a new normal. Patience isn't just a virtue here - it's mandatory.

Sometimes, though, you need to bring in the professionals. Watch for red flags like sudden loss of sex drive, pain during sex, extreme mood swings, unexplained weight changes, or constant fatigue. These could signal deeper issues that need expert attention. Don't be afraid to consult a hormone specialist, sex therapist, relationship counselor, or functional medicine doctor. Getting help isn't admitting defeat - it's being smart enough to know when you're out of your depth.

Fixing a low sex drive isn't about miracle pills or quick fixes. It's about creating an environment where desire can flourish naturally. Get stress under control. Fix those hormone imbalances. Clean up your diet and get moving together. Build a real emotional connection. Most importantly, have some patience. A watched pot never boils, and a pressured partner never gets horny. Focus on improving her life, and the bedroom situation will follow suit.

If all this seems overwhelming, remember even small changes can lead to big results. Start with one thing. It could be taking over kid duty one night a week so she can have alone time. It could be cleaning up your diet together. Pick something, stick with it, and build from there.

Chapter 4: Having a Sex Life with Kids In the House

We've all been there. You're about to get it on for the first time in weeks. The mood is perfect. Your partner's giving you that look. Then – BAM! – tiny footsteps in the hallway. "Daddy, I had a bad dream..." Game over. Sound familiar?

If you're nodding your head right now, choking back bitter laughter while remembering your own cockblocked moments, keep reading. This isn't another sugarcoated "parenting expert" chapter telling you to find your zen. This is about getting your sex life back from the tiny terrorists who've taken it hostage.

Since the kids came along, getting laid has become harder than quantum physics. But before we get into the battle plan for getting sex life back, we need to talk about what your woman's been through.

Now, this is important. Your lady just pushed a whole human being out of her body. Her vagina's been through D-Day, her hormones are more messed up than a meth lab explosion, and her tits have gone from fun bags to food dispensers. Could you imagine somebody putting your balls in a vice for nine months, then expecting you to be horny right after?

She's not avoiding sex because she doesn't want you anymore. She's avoiding it because her body has been through a war. She's getting woken up every two hours by a screaming machine that's literally sucking the life out of her tits. Romance isn't exactly top of mind when you're leaking milk through your shirt and haven't slept more than three consecutive hours in months.

So here's what you're going to do: Be supportive. Your job right now is to be her rock. Hold her when she cries for no reason. Take the baby so she can shower in peace. Clean the house without expecting anything in return. The more supported she feels now, the faster she'll get back to feeling like a woman.

Now, once you pass that initial "holy sh*t, we have a baby" phase and into your new life as parents, that is the time you can start thinking about your sex life again. That spark isn't dead; it's just buried under a mountain of diapers, sleep deprivation, and baby puke. Time to dig it out and remind yourselves what sex was before you were Mom and Dad.

Sleep Training the Baby

Welcome to Boot Camp: Operation Get Some. We're going to whip your kids' sleep habits into shape so you can remember what your woman looks like naked.

Step one: Identify. Every kid's got their own messed up sleep sabotage strategy. Is your little angel a midnight marathon runner or a 3 AM opera singer? Figure out their tactics like you're planning a covert op.

Next, choose your battle plan. Are you going hard with the "Cry It Out" method or softie with "No Tears?" It doesn't matter; just pick one and stick to it like your sex life depends on it - because it does.

Consistency is key. Your kid is going to test you like you're in basic training. Don't break. You're tougher than a sleep-deprived toddler... barely.

Now, create a bedtime routine tighter than your college drinking schedule. Bath, book, bed - no negotiations. You're the general of this army.

Once you've got the little terrorist down, it's go time. Your mission: Reconnect with that smoking hot babe you love before she forgets what your face looks like. Start small. Maybe actually finish a conversation without baby crying. Or hell, crazy idea - touch each other without a kid wedged between you like a chastity belt.

With a solid sleep training plan, you'll be back to taking care of your lady in the sack in no time - just like the good old days!

Timing When to Have Sex

Timing is everything when you're trying to get it on as parents. You need to get strategic like you're planning a heist. Your new best friend? The kids' schedule. Nap time isn't just for catching up on your Instagram feed anymore; it's prime time for you and your woman. Set the alarm, be ready to sprint back to the bedroom like Usain Bolt, and be sure to make those precious minutes count before the tiny man or woman wakes up.

Speaking of energy, you aren't that endless stamina machine you used to be back in college, and neither is your lady. By the time those little humans finally pass out, you're both ready to face-plant harder than a drunk at last call. Here's your solution: mornings. Set that alarm 30 minutes early and start your day by satisfying your woman. You'll be amazed how sex first thing in the morning can energize your whole day.

Weekends? That's your time to shine, but you have to be strategic. Take turns with the little ones: one day, you handle them, and the next day, she does. Whoever gets to sleep in is responsible for initiating.

Learn to love quickies. Ten minutes of action in the laundry room while cartoons hypnotize the kids can be gold for your relationship.

Too tired to try? Time to get creative. Mutual masturbation just became your new favorite hobby: quick, dirty, and gets the job done. Plus, watching your lady pleasure herself while you stroke yourself can be hot and remind you both why you couldn't keep your hands off each other before the kids came along.

Stay in the game. Send her sexy texts while the kids are in school. Grab her butt when she's loading the dishwasher, and whisper nasty things into her ear during family movie night. That keeps her engine revving for when you finally get a chance.

Just remember, your sex life is about keeping that fire with your woman. That sometimes means choosing between pleasing her and catching those precious Zs. In that case, always please her! Yeah, you will be a zombie the next day, but you are a satisfied zombie, and so is she.

And the truth about scheduling sex is that it sounds like the opposite of a flourishing sex life. But having that appointment on the calendar builds anticipation like a horny teenager. It gives you both time to prepare.

There's your blueprint. With a bit of planning and some great attitude, you can keep the intimacy, even with a house full of tiny cockblockers.

How to Deal With the Older Kids

It's a massive challenge having sex with older kids in the house. Every creak of the bed, every groan, every outburst of passion has got to be planned like a Special Forces operation.

The brutal truth that few will admit is that your sex life is, in fact, one of the main ingredients in preventing your family from falling apart. It's holding together the base of your entire household. It's crucial for you and your lady.

First order of business, you need boundaries thicker than steel. Your sex life needs to be tighter than Fort Knox. With kids under 10, you say bedtime is bedtime-period. The beauty is those hours after they fall asleep.

And now, about stealth mode: White noise machines aren't just for babies; they're to drown out Mommy and Daddy's special wrestling time. Get a good fan, crank up the music, whatever it takes. And remember to invest in some quality door locks. Nothing kills the mood as much as tiny hands turning doorknobs at the worst possible moment.

If the worst happens, and your child catches you while doing it, here's how you handle it: keep cool, explain that this is private adult time, and then move on as though nothing happened.

So, no feeling guilty about wanting to make your sex life flourish with kids at home. It is actually the opposite. If there is intimacy, both of you will be better parents.

Chapter 5: Long-Term Sex Life Strategies

So, I hope some of the strategies in the previous chapters will help you get your sex life back, but how do you make it last and not fall back into some dead bedroom situation again? Time for advanced-level sex life strategies.

Think of your sex life like this: use it or lose it. It's about keeping that sexual engine hot for the long haul. Step in the "don't break the chain" method from Jerry Seinfeld's playbook.

How it works: every time you have sex, put a big X on the calendar. The goal is not to let that string of Xs break. This is not some wild suggestion; this is your new life. It's about making sure sex is a natural part of your life instead of becoming some distant memory.

Now, here's where stuff gets interesting: the Sex Life Bucket List. This is your sex script waiting to happen. Sit down with your partner and get nasty with your imagination. What kind of filthy things have you both been dreaming about? Maybe she wants to get away for a weekend in some fancy hotel, or perhaps you want her to dress like a naughty nurse. Those random "Wouldn't it be hot if..." thoughts you get while driving around? Put those on the list. That scene that made her as wet as Niagara Falls? Put that on, too.

But what's magical about this list is not just crossing things off. It's all about the anticipation, the planning, the dirty talk about what you will do to each other. It keeps the sexual tension simmering.

Keep in mind, this isn't about becoming some tantric sex guru or porn star- not unless that is already on your bucket list. It's about keeping your sex life active and investing in each other's fantasies. Stay consistent, add to that bucket list, and never break the chain. You will be thankful.

Sex Bucket List Ideas

Fantasies are like mental Viagra, and it's time to pop that pill. It's time to level up your sex game. Here are some ideas to get you and your partner's mental juices flowing. You have been warned: this is not the plain missionary position.

Create sensations that will have her squirming. Blindfolds take away one sense to ramp up others. Bringing yourselves to the brink and backing off builds tension until you both go off.

Get into power play.

Be in control one night and get out the paddle or handcuffs if that's your thing. The next time, you will be at her mercy. Switching roles keeps things exciting and helps you better understand each other's preferences. Just establish safe words and boundaries first.

Speaking of boundaries, let's talk about the back door.

Anal play isn't for everyone, but if you are both curious, start slow. Use lots of lube, patience, and maybe some toys to warm up. Rimming, plugs -there's a whole world of sensation to explore if you're ready for it. The prostate can provide mind-blowing orgasms for guys open to exploring.

Give her an erotic massage using scented oils. Take the time to find every sensitive spot. Learn where the G-spot is and how to work it. Pay attention to the clitoris - it's the command center of her pleasures. Different angles, pressures, rhythms, and stimulating it with various toys.

Get creative with grooming. Variable lengths and shapes of the pubic hair bring in new sensations. Try fully clothed sex. Practice naked yoga together: flexibility and intimacy go hand in hand.

Want to push the envelope? Have a sex party or invite another person into your bed. This isn't for everybody and needs honest communication and trust. Make sure all participants are comfortable and that a few ground rules are clearly made. Nothing ruins a good time like jealousy or misunderstandings.

Read erotica together; it's like porn for the brain. It gives you a chance to work out your fantasies safely before trying them in reality. Roleplay these fantasies: dress up, create a scenario, and let your imagination go wild. That strict teacher fantasy? Yep, it's time to make it a reality.

Stock up on a selection of condoms: ribbed, ultra-thin, and warming lube. Yes, you're in a committed relationship, but a change in sensation is a pleasant added surprise. Just make sure to test it on a small area first. Chemical burns on your junk are sure to kill the mood.

And finally, make your list. These are just suggestions to get you started. The best erotic adventures are those that you'll discover together.

Couples who talk about sex have more sex. Sharing fantasies is like getting to level two of your relationship game. This isn't about heating things in your bedroom but getting vulnerable. Create a safe space where judgment is not an option. If she says something you think is weird, don't laugh. Instead, ask questions, listen, and be curious.

Lastly, seek professional help. If you're struggling, hire a pro: A sex therapist or coach

can give you tips catered to your own needs.
Just remember: keeping your sex life lit over the
long run is not about putting sex on a pedestal;
it's the opposite. Do all you can to make sex a
regular activity in your relationship.

Chapter 6: Sex Life Tips for Men

Time to talk about sex - real sex. Not the Hollywood version, not the porn fantasy, not some young buck's highlight reel, but the kind of sex that keeps a long-term relationship smoking hot.

Almost 30% of women need a little bit more than penetration to hit the peak. That is not a weakness; that is an easy way for you to become a sex god. You have your hands, your mouth, and, yeah, your dick. That's a full arsenal of pleasure tools at your disposal. The average guy stops at penetration and wonders why she's not screaming his name.

Foreplay is where you get to be the man. Building up pleasure is like an orchestra, and you're the conductor. Her body's got multiple instruments to play- why would you only use one? The real magic happens when you learn to work all her sweet spots together. That's when you become the lover she brags about to her friends.

Remember: Any good craftsman knows how to use every tool in his toolbox. The great lover utilizes everything in his power to drive her wild.

Stop trying to guess what gets her off. Ask her. "You like that?" "Tell me what you want," "Show me how you touch yourself." And when she's telling you? Listen up. If she says "right there," don't move a muscle except when she tells you to. A woman who feels heard in the bedroom will let loose in ways that blow your mind. That means actually listening to her responses, both verbal and physical.

Sex begins in the brain, so if her head's not into it, neither will her body.

Here's what works: a fresh shower, clean sheets, and a bedroom that's ready for action. It's not complicated, but it sets the stage for what will happen. When your space is prepared, she can focus on what matters—pleasure.

Great sex is about both of you losing your minds together. It's a skill, and as with any other skill, it takes practice, attention, and real effort if you are going to master it. Take your time. Pay attention to her signals. Be present. It is not a sprint to the finish line.

Make Her Cum

Women want a man who can read their body like a map. You need to be present and focused. Make her feel like she's the only woman in existence. Every moan, every grab, every arch of her back is telling you something.

Want to take it to the next level with missionary? The coital alignment technique.

Basically, ride higher up so that your dick is rubbing on her clit with every stroke. Slow, deep strokes, grinding on her, that's where it's at. Let her ride you, cowgirl, and she can grind that clit on your pelvis until she explodes. The lotus position? Same thing, it is all about that clit contact while you're deep inside her.

Now, let's get into eating kitty. This is your chance to make her cum harder than she ever has before. Get in there and pay attention to how she moves against your mouth. When she starts grinding on your face, follow her lead. That means she's telling you precisely what she needs. Mix it up with your tongue, fingers, and lips, but when she's close, you better not change one single thing you're doing. Keep that same rhythm until she's shaking.

And don't sleep on making out, either. Deep, passionate kissing floods her body with feel-good chemicals that get her horny as hell. Kiss her neck, bite her ears, grab her shoulders- all those spots can drive her wild. This isn't just foreplay; this is part of getting her whole body ready to explode.

Now, on to the more advanced territory: her butt. Her cheeks are packed with nerve endings that can send electricity through her whole body. Grab it, squeeze it, spank it. Some women love their butt played with; others don't.

And the biggest no-no of all: overthinking. Keep it real. Focus on what's making her moan right now. Pay attention to how wet she's getting. Listen for her breathing change when you hit the right spot. That's the way to make her come harder than she ever has before. But the endgame isn't just to make her come; it's to have sex so good she does not remember her name, which also includes afterplay.

Afterplay

Don't commit the sin of rolling over and passing out or immediately jumping straight onto your phone after she has had a mind-blowing orgasm. This is prime time for creating super strong sexual bonds. How you handle afterplay will significantly impact keeping that spark lit over the long term. Here are three things you can try.

The Talk-It-Out Types

Sometimes, you might want to debrief after your brains get screwed. Maybe you tried something new and kinky, or she came harder than ever before. This is gold for your sex game-you're getting real-time feedback on what worked and what didn't. I'm not saying you should be making it weird with a full-on interview, but "That thing you did with your hips? F*cking incredible" can go a long way.

Pro Tip: Ask her what part she will be thinking about tomorrow. Plant that seed in her head that she will be replaying all day.

The Silent Assassins

Sometimes, words just totally ruin the vibe. If you just had earth-shattering sex, lying there in comfortable silence can be powerful. Of course, this is when you have that deep connection and don't need to say anything to know what's up with each other.

Pro tip: Make a deal to stay completely quiet for a few minutes, just holding each other. It's more intense than you'd think.

The Pass-Out Crew

There's nothing wrong if you want to sleep immediately after an intense session that drained your tanks. Sex is great for getting quality sleep. Those hormones are better than any sleeping pill.

Pro tip: Pull her close and match your breathing. It's intimate and will have you both sleeping like babies.

Authors' note

If you've read this far, I hope I've given you something worth your time and attention. But before we end, let's look at what three different couples have done to start sleeping with each other again.

Case Study 1: Rekindling Love After Empty Nest

Last month, I ran into Julius and Meghan at a couple's therapy conference in Denver. They were two people in their late 50s, married for 32 years, looking more like awkward high schoolers on a first date than a couple who'd raised three kids together. They were there as success stories, but six months earlier... a totally different story.

"We hadn't had sex in almost two years," Julius admitted over coffee, wincing like he was confessing to a crime. "Hell, we barely touched each other anymore. Just two strangers sharing a mortgage and memories of when we used to bang like rabbits."

Meghan, this fierce freespirited grandmother of two, rolled her eyes at her husband's bluntness but nodded. "After the kids moved out, we realized we'd forgotten how to be lovers. We knew how to be parents, how to run a household, but actually wanting each other? That felt like ancient history."

The breaking point came during a Sunday dinner when their youngest daughter, now a psych major, bluntly asked why they never showed affection anymore. Talk about getting called out by your own kid. That night, they had their first real conversation about sex in years, and it wasn't pretty.

"I felt like a failure as a woman," Meghan confessed, tears welling up. "My body had changed, and I couldn't remember the last time I felt sexy." Julius jumped in: "And I was scared to initiate anything. Rejection at this age? Man, that's a whole 'nother beast."

But here's where it gets good. Instead of letting their dead bedroom become their new normal, they got help. Found this amazing sex therapist who didn't sugarcoat anything. First session, she looked them dead in the eye and said, "Your marriage isn't dying. Your comfort zone is killing it."

The homework started simple: Five minutes of eye contact every night. No phones, no TV, just looking at each other. "It was awkward," Julius laughed. "But by week two, something shifted. I started seeing my wife again, not just the mother of my kids."

They graduated to non-sexual touch. Massages, hand-holding, dancing in the kitchen. Meghan started booking regular salon appointments, not for Julius, but because it made her feel good. Julius hit the gym, not to get ripped, but to feel stronger, more confident.

Three months in, they had sex for the first time in years. "It wasn't perfect," Meghan grinned, "but it was real. Raw. Honest." Julius couldn't stop smiling: "We'd forgotten how to play, how to flirt. Now we're like school kids again, but with better technique and more stamina."

Today? They're that annoying couple who can't keep their hands off each other at family gatherings. Their kids pretend to be grossed out, but secretly? They're taking notes.

"Look," Julius said, finishing his third espresso, "we almost let our marriage die of boredom. But here's the truth: great sex after 50 isn't about trying to recreate what worked at 30. It's about building something new, something honest, something that fits who you are now."

Meghan's parting shot? "And invest in good lube. Lots of it. That's non-negotiable after menopause."

Their success wasn't just about getting back in the bedroom - it was about completely redefining intimacy at their age. They created what they call their "Second Honeymoon Handbook," a set of rules and rituals that worked for who they are now, not who they were thirty years ago.

"We had to learn that foreplay isn't just physical anymore," Meghan explained, stirring her tea. "It's about emotional connection. Sometimes it starts with morning texts, or the way Julius looks at me across a room full of people. The anticipation builds all day."

They also had to navigate some uniquely middle-aged challenges. Their youngest moved back home temporarily after college, which threw a wrench in their newfound freedom. "Try explaining why the kitchen counter needs to be disinfected at 2 PM," Julius chuckled. "We had to get creative with timing and location again, just like when the kids were little."

The physical aspects required some adjustments too. They invested in a high-end mattress for joint comfort, kept water and snacks handy for energy, and weren't shy about using aids when needed. "Our generation didn't talk about this stuff," Meghan said. "But now? I'll march right into that adult store and ask questions. No shame in our game."

Their friends started noticing the change. Some asked for advice, others seemed uncomfortable with their obvious affection. "We lost a couple of dinner party invites," Julius admitted. "Apparently, it makes some people uncomfortable when you're still hot for each other at our age. Their loss."

The most unexpected benefit was how their renewed intimacy affected other areas of their life. They started making better health choices, not because their doctor nagged them, but because they wanted to keep their sex life active. They communicated better about everything, not just bedroom matters. Even their financial planning improved - they started prioritizing experiences over things.

"You know what people don't tell you about sex after 50?" Meghan leaned in, lowering her voice. "It can actually be better than when you're young. You know your body, you know your partner, and you're not trying to impress anyone. Plus, the kids are grown, and you can afford decent wine."

Julius nodded enthusiastically. "And hotel rooms. Don't forget spontaneous hotel rooms in the middle of the week just because we can. Try doing that when you're young with a mortgage and soccer practice."

Now they're that couple who gives hope to others their age. They mentor other couples through their church's marriage ministry, sharing their story with brutal honesty and practical advice. "The number one thing we tell people?" Meghan said, squeezing Julius's hand. "It's never too late to start over. Never too late to fall in love again. And definitely never too late for great sex."

The real gold in their story isn't just that they got their groove back — it's how they completely rewrote their relationship playbook. Let me break down exactly how they went from "dead bedroom" to "get a room" in their late 50s.

First up, they had to face some uncomfortable truths. Meghan spent an entire therapy session ugly-crying about how she'd catch glimpses of herself in the mirror and didn't recognize the woman looking back. "I kept comparing myself to the 28-year-old Julius married," she admitted. "That woman could rock a bikini and stay up all night. This version of me needs reading glasses to check her phone and has joints that crack like bubble wrap."

Julius had his own demons to wrestle. "I was dealing with some occasional ED issues but was too proud to talk about it. Instead, I just stopped initiating. Easier to watch Sports Center than risk not being able to perform." Their therapist hit them with some real talk: They were letting pride and fear cock-block their happiness.

The turning point came during what they call "The Great Lingerie Disaster of 2023." Meghan, trying to spice things up, ordered some fancy underwear online. "I looked like a stuffed sausage trying to escape its casing," she laughed. "But instead of crying about it, I walked out to show Julius anyway. Just owned it." Julius's reaction? "She looked f*cking gorgeous because she was trying. That vulnerability was sexier than any piece of overpriced lace."

They started treating their relationship like a project that needed daily attention. Every morning, they'd spend 15 minutes just touching – not groping or trying to get it on, but actually connecting physically. "Sometimes it was just holding hands while drinking coffee. Other times it was a shoulder massage. The point was making physical contact a normal part of our day again," Julius explained.

Their sex therapist gave them homework that would make most couples their age blush. They had to create a "Yes/No/Maybe" list of sexual activities they wanted to try. "That list saved our sex life," Meghan declared. "Turns out Julius had some kinky ideas he'd been sitting on for thirty years, and I had some fantasies I'd never admitted to anyone."

The breakthrough wasn't just about getting naked more often. It was about getting real with each other. They started having what they call "naked truth sessions" where they'd literally strip down and talk about their fears, desires, and insecurities. "There's something about being physically naked that makes it easier to be emotionally naked too," Meghan reflected.

They also had to deal with the physical realities of sex after 50. "Lube became our best friend," Julius chuckled. "And we learned that sometimes you need to plan ahead. If we know we want to get intimate, we both take it easy at dinner, maybe pop a vitamin, make sure we're well-rested. It's not as spontaneous as it used to be, but who cares? The orgasms are better."

The kids noticed the change in their relationship before they even said anything. Their oldest son actually pulled Julius aside at a family barbecue: "Dad, whatever you and Mom are doing, keep it up. You guys seem really happy." Talk about validation.

But it wasn't all smooth sailing. They had setbacks. Meghan went through a rough patch during menopause that put sex off the table for a few weeks. Instead of letting it derail their progress, they focused on other forms of intimacy. "We took baths together, gave each other massages, made out like teenagers. Kept that connection alive even when penetrative sex wasn't an option," Julius shared.

They also had to redefine what "good sex" meant at this stage of life. "In our 30s, it was all about how many times we could do it in one night," Meghan explained. "Now it's about quality over quantity. We might only have sex once a week, but it lasts longer, feels more connected, and honestly? The orgasms are way better because we actually know what we're doing."

Their new approach to intimacy spilled over into other areas of their life. They started taking dance classes together and planned regular weekend getaway. "It's like we're dating again, but with three decades of inside jokes and shared history to build on," Julius grinned.

The biggest lesson they learned? Great sex after 50 isn't about trying to recreate your youth – it's about creating something new that works for who you are now. "We're not trying to compete with our younger selves," Meghan insisted. "We're creating our own rules, our own definition of sexy, and honestly? It feels better than ever."

Case Study 2: Finding Love in the Wildness of Family Life

Darren was already running late for his son's basketball game when his wife Tiana hit him with it: "When was the last time we actually had sex?" She wasn't being accusatory. Just stating facts while loading their youngest into the minivan. Four kids, two careers, and a sex life that had become as rare as a quiet Sunday morning.

"Man, that question haunted me through the whole game," Darren told me over beers months later. "I couldn't even remember. That's when I knew we had a serious problem."

Let me paint you the full picture: Darren, 42, successful architect, coaching youth basketball on weekends. Tiana, 39, pediatric nurse working night shifts three times a week. Four kids aged 4 to 12, all in different activities. Their calendar looked like a game of Tetris played by a caffeine-addicted squirrel.

The challenges were relentless. Darren's architecture firm had him juggling three major projects, often requiring late-night revisions. Tiana's night shifts meant she slept during the day when Darren was most energetic. Their oldest had soccer three times a week, the middle two were in competitive swimming, and the youngest had just started dance classes. Every minute seemed scheduled, double-booked, or spent recovering from the last activity.

"We were like two ships passing in the night," Tiana explained. "I'd get home from my shift just as he was leaving for work. By the time we were both home, there were homework battles, dinner mess, and someone always needed something."

Even when they had a moment alone, exhaustion took over. They'd tried the occasional date night, but they were both so tired they'd end up just talking about the kids or falling asleep at the restaurant. Physical intimacy had become an afterthought, something they'd get to "when things calmed down." But things never calmed down.

The breaking point came during a rare quiet moment when they both realized they couldn't remember the last time they'd been intimate. No drama, no fighting, just that stark realization that they'd become excellent co-parents and terrible lovers.

Their solution started with an honest late-night conversation. After listing every obstacle — from Tiana's erratic work schedule to Darren's project deadlines, from their youngest's habit of crawling into their bed at 2 AM to their complete lack of energy management – they created an intimacy plan.

First, they tackled the scheduling nightmare. Tiana negotiated with her hospital supervisor to switch to predominantly day shifts, even though it meant a 15% pay cut. "We did the math," Darren explained. "The loss in income was worth it compared to the cost of couples therapy or, worse, divorce." They also hired a regular babysitter for Wednesday evenings, not for fancy date nights, but just to have guaranteed adult time in their own home.

The physical space needed work too. Their master bedroom had become a family gathering spot, with kids' toys scattered everywhere and no real privacy. They invested in proper locks, moved the kids' gaming console to the basement, and established clear boundaries about their private space. "We even installed a mini-fridge in our room," Tiana shared.

"Sounds silly, but not having to go downstairs for water meant one less reason to break the mood."

Their morning strategy became crucial. "We started waking up an hour before the kids," Tiana shared. "Sometimes we'd have sex, sometimes we'd just talk or shower together. But that time became sacred." They set up a traffic light system outside their door. Green meant kids could knock, red meant wait unless the house was literally on fire.

The household management overhaul was next. They audited every task that ate into their energy and time. Grocery shopping? Switched to delivery. Lawn care? Hired a service. House cleaning? Brought in bi-weekly help. They taught their older kids to do their own laundry and implemented a strict "everyone cleans their own mess" policy.

"The energy management was crucial," Darren explained. "We realized we were spending our best hours on everything except our relationship." They started treating their intimate time like any other important appointment. They blocked out specific times in their shared calendar, complete with preparation time. "If you're exhausted by 9 PM, scheduling 'sexy time' for 10 PM is just setting yourself up for failure," Tiana noted.

They developed a sophisticated system of signals and codes for initiating sex without broadcasting it to the whole house. A specific emoji in a text message. A certain way of touching while passing in the hallway. Tiana would wear particular earrings when she was feeling sexy; Darren had his "lucky" blue shirt that signaled his interest.

"We also had to address the mental barriers," Darren admitted. "I was carrying work stress home, checking emails until bedtime. Tiana was constantly in 'mom mode.' We had to learn to transition between our roles." They created decompression rituals. Darren would take a 10-minute walk after work before entering the house, Tiana would do quick meditation between her shift and family time.

The physical intimacy rebuild was gradual. They started with a "touch quota." The minimal daily physical contact that didn't have to lead to sex. Morning hugs, casual touches, proper kisses instead of quick pecks. "We had to remind our bodies that we were lovers, not just co-parents," Tiana explained.

They also got practical about spontaneity. "We realized waiting for the perfect moment was killing our sex life," Darren said. "So we created perfect moments." They kept essential items in strategic locations, maintained backup plans for interruptions, and learned to take advantage of small windows of opportunity.

Six months into their new approach, they're having sex at least twice a week. A miracle by busy parent standards. But more importantly, they've rediscovered their connection as partners, not just co-parents. Their system isn't perfect. Kids still interrupt, work still gets crazy, and sometimes they're just too tired. But now they have a framework for getting back on track.

Their advice to other parents drowning in family life is: "Stop waiting for the perfect moment," Tiana insisted. "Create it. Protect it. Fight for it if you have to. And remember that your relationship needs infrastructure just like any other important part of your life."

Darren added: "And remember, you're not just parents. You're lovers who happened to create a family together. Don't lose that part of yourselves. It takes work, planning, and sometimes a really good lock on your bedroom door."

Their story proves that reviving intimacy in a busy family isn't about grand gestures or dramatic changes. It's about creating systems, establishing boundaries, and making your relationship a priority in practical, sustainable ways.

Case Study 3: From Power Couple to Powerless Passion

I met Alex and Jamie at a burnout recovery retreat in Sedona last fall. Picture two high-powered New York executives, both 33, looking like they'd just crawled out of the corporate trenches. Alex, investment banker, hadn't slept more than four hours straight in months. Jamie, consultant, was mainlining espresso like it was oxygen.

"We were that couple everyone envied on Instagram," Jamie told me over sunrise yoga. "Great careers, luxury apartment, exotic vacations. But behind closed doors? We hadn't had sex in three months. We were too exhausted to even fight about it."

Alex nodded, his Rolex catching the morning light. "Last time we tried, I literally fell asleep during foreplay. Jamie was checking work emails while giving me a handjob. That's when we knew we'd hit rock bottom."

Their story is classic Manhattan power couple sh*t. Met at Harvard Business School, both graduated top of their class, got married after a whirlwind romance. Sex used to be their stress relief. Quickies in the office after hours, luxury hotel getaways, the works. Then success hit like a freight train.

"We were crushing it professionally," Alex explained during our follow-up dinner in the city. "But something had to give, and it was our sex life."

Their wake-up call came during a board meeting, of all places. Jamie was presenting quarterly projections when she suddenly burst into tears. Not cute movie tears – full-on ugly crying in front of twelve associates. "I looked at these graphs showing our company's growth, and all I could think was how my relationship was going in the opposite direction."

The next day, they had their first real conversation in months. No phones, no laptops, just two people finally admitting they were drowning in success and dying in their relationship.

"We laid it all out," Alex shared. "The 80-hour weeks. The sleeping pills. The porn addiction I'd developed because it was easier than trying to initiate sex when we were both exhausted. The fact that Jamie had been faking orgasms for months just to get it over with faster."

Instead of just throwing money at the problem with fancy couples retreats or sex therapy (though they did that too), they decided to completely restructure their lives. First move? They both set hard boundaries at work.

"I told my associates I'd be offline from 7 PM to 7 AM unless the company was literally on fire," Jamie said. "They weren't happy, but f*ck it my marriage was more important than their midnight email anxiety."

Alex took it a step further, dropping to four days a week at the firm. One day remote. "Yeah, it cost me some bonus potential. But you know what's more expensive? Divorce."

They created a detox protocol." No phones in the bedroom. No work calls during dinner. And most importantly, no more using their Type A personalities as an excuse to avoid intimacy.

"We had to learn how to turn off our business brains," Jamie explained. "Do you know how hard it is for two overachievers to stop treating sex like a performance review? I literally caught myself making a spreadsheet to track our orgasms."

Alex chimed in, loosening his tie: "I had to unlearn everything I thought made me successful. That constant need to be 'on,' to be performing, to be in control. It was killing our bedroom chemistry. Turns out you can't PowerPoint your way into better sex."

They hired a sex coach who specialized in working with executives. First session, she made them do something radical: spend an entire weekend together with no agenda. No scheduled activities, no restaurant reservations, no planned sex.

"It was terrifying," Jamie admitted. "Two control freaks with no schedule? I almost had a panic attack. But by Sunday, we'd remembered how to just... be together. We ended up having sex in our shower. Something we hadn't done since business school."

The real breakthrough came when they started treating their sex life with the same strategic thinking they applied to their careers but in reverse. Instead of maximizing and optimizing, they focused on minimizing and simplifying.

"We created 'desire windows,'" Alex explained. "Times when we both committed to being available and present. No pressure to perform, just... space for possibility. Sometimes we'd just make out. Sometimes we'd f*ck like porn stars. The point was creating the opportunity."

They also had to address their individual issues. Jamie had been using work as an excuse to avoid dealing with body image issues that crept in after years of stress eating at her desk. Alex had to confront how his porn habit had warped his expectations of real intimacy.

"The hardest part?" Jamie leaned in, lowering her voice. "Learning that great sex doesn't always look like a highlight reel. Sometimes it's messy. Sometimes it's quick. Sometimes one of us doesn't finish, and that's okay. We had to stop treating our sex life like another metric to optimize."

"We also had to learn how to fight fair about sex," Alex noted. "No more passive-aggressive comments about being too tired. No more using work as a weapon. If one of us is feeling neglected, we say it directly."

Six months in, they're having sex three to four times a week – quality sex, not just checking-a-box sex. More importantly, they've found a sustainable balance between their ambitious careers and their need for intimacy.

"Here's what no one tells you about success," Jamie reflected, swirling her wine. "You can have the corner office, the seven-figure bonus, and mind-blowing sex – but not if you're trying to maximize everything all the time. Something's got to give, and it shouldn't be your relationship."

Their advice to other power couples? "Stop treating your relationship like another project to manage," Alex insisted. "Your partner isn't a quarterly target or a client to impress. They're your safe space from all that bullsh*t."

Jamie's final thought? "And, stop bringing your phone to bed. Nothing kills desire faster than checking Bloomberg while your partner's trying to go down on you."

Today, they're still crushing it professionally, but with boundaries that protect their connection. They've become that rare species in Manhattan: a power couple that actually has power over their own lives.

"We're not perfect," Jamie admitted. "Sometimes work still wins. But now we know how to find our way back to each other. And honestly, the sex is better when you're not trying to optimize it like a spreadsheet."

Final words on how to make it work again

My goal with this book was to make sex a regular part of your relationship again. Do you think I've delivered on that? Please tell me in the reviews or rate the book so other readers know what to expect.

But before we end, let's repeat the truth of what women want and what's the foundation for relationship success that will have the most significant impact on your sex life.

Mental Toughness: Having uncomfortable conversations. Admitting when you're wrong. Listening instead of waiting for your turn to talk.

Emotional Intelligence: Understanding your baggage. Learning your partner's emotional language. Dealing with your shit instead of dumping it on her. Being vulnerable without being weak.

Physical Presence: Being there when it's inconvenient. Making time when there isn't any. Creating moments instead of waiting for them.

And remember: this is the beginning of the new normal—a new normal in which sex is a regular thing in your relationship again. Thanks for reading!

Contact me:

Any questions, concerns about the books or ideas for new books you want to share? Please email me at: adamlewisbooks@gmail.com

Or sign up for my readers team. It's free; you get audiobook coupon codes, free books (before they are published), and much more! https://bit.ly/3ZvdEz8

* 9 7 8 9 1 9 8 9 8 9 5 8 8 *